MEDICAL APPOINTMENT TRACKER

THIS BOOK BELONGS TO:

_____

_____

_____

_____

Copyright © 2020 MPX2 Publishing Company
All Rights Reserved

DATE	TIME	DOCTOR		CONTACT
REASON FOR VISIT		QUESTIONS		OUTCOME
				MEDICATION PERSCRIBED
NOTES				TREATMENT
				FOLLOW UP

DATE	TIME	DOCTOR		CONTACT
REASON FOR VISIT		QUESTIONS		OUTCOME
				MEDICATION PERSCRIBED
NOTES				TREATMENT
				FOLLOW UP

DATE	TIME	DOCTOR		CONTACT
REASON FOR VISIT		QUESTIONS		OUTCOME
				MEDICATION PERSCRIBED
NOTES				TREATMENT
				FOLLOW UP

DATE	TIME	DOCTOR	CONTACT
REASON FOR VISIT		QUESTIONS	OUTCOME
			MEDICATION PERSCRIBED
NOTES			TREATMENT
			FOLLOW UP

DATE	TIME	DOCTOR	CONTACT
REASON FOR VISIT		QUESTIONS	OUTCOME
			MEDICATION PERSCRIBED
NOTES			TREATMENT
			FOLLOW UP

DATE	TIME	DOCTOR	CONTACT
REASON FOR VISIT		QUESTIONS	OUTCOME
			MEDICATION PERSCRIBED
NOTES			TREATMENT
			FOLLOW UP

DATE	TIME	DOCTOR		CONTACT
REASON FOR VISIT		QUESTIONS		OUTCOME
				MEDICATION PERSCRIBED
NOTES				TREATMENT
				FOLLOW UP

DATE	TIME	DOCTOR		CONTACT
REASON FOR VISIT		QUESTIONS		OUTCOME
				MEDICATION PERSCRIBED
NOTES				TREATMENT
				FOLLOW UP

DATE	TIME	DOCTOR		CONTACT
REASON FOR VISIT		QUESTIONS		OUTCOME
				MEDICATION PERSCRIBED
NOTES				TREATMENT
				FOLLOW UP

DATE	TIME	DOCTOR		CONTACT
REASON FOR VISIT		QUESTIONS		OUTCOME
				MEDICATION PERSCRIBED
NOTES				TREATMENT
				FOLLOW UP

DATE	TIME	DOCTOR		CONTACT
REASON FOR VISIT		QUESTIONS		OUTCOME
				MEDICATION PERSCRIBED
NOTES				TREATMENT
				FOLLOW UP

DATE	TIME	DOCTOR		CONTACT
REASON FOR VISIT		QUESTIONS		OUTCOME
				MEDICATION PERSCRIBED
NOTES				TREATMENT
				FOLLOW UP

DATE	TIME	DOCTOR		CONTACT
REASON FOR VISIT		QUESTIONS		OUTCOME
				MEDICATION PERSCRIBED
NOTES				TREATMENT
				FOLLOW UP

DATE	TIME	DOCTOR		CONTACT
REASON FOR VISIT		QUESTIONS		OUTCOME
				MEDICATION PERSCRIBED
NOTES				TREATMENT
				FOLLOW UP

DATE	TIME	DOCTOR		CONTACT
REASON FOR VISIT		QUESTIONS		OUTCOME
				MEDICATION PERSCRIBED
NOTES				TREATMENT
				FOLLOW UP

DATE	TIME	DOCTOR		CONTACT
REASON FOR VISIT		QUESTIONS		OUTCOME
				MEDICATION PERSCRIBED
NOTES				TREATMENT
				FOLLOW UP

DATE	TIME	DOCTOR		CONTACT
REASON FOR VISIT		QUESTIONS		OUTCOME
				MEDICATION PERSCRIBED
NOTES				TREATMENT
				FOLLOW UP

DATE	TIME	DOCTOR		CONTACT
REASON FOR VISIT		QUESTIONS		OUTCOME
				MEDICATION PERSCRIBED
NOTES				TREATMENT
				FOLLOW UP

DATE	TIME	DOCTOR		CONTACT
REASON FOR VISIT		QUESTIONS		OUTCOME
				MEDICATION PERSCRIBED
NOTES				TREATMENT
				FOLLOW UP

DATE	TIME	DOCTOR		CONTACT
REASON FOR VISIT		QUESTIONS		OUTCOME
				MEDICATION PERSCRIBED
NOTES				TREATMENT
				FOLLOW UP

DATE	TIME	DOCTOR		CONTACT
REASON FOR VISIT		QUESTIONS		OUTCOME
				MEDICATION PERSCRIBED
NOTES				TREATMENT
				FOLLOW UP

DATE	TIME	DOCTOR	CONTACT
REASON FOR VISIT		QUESTIONS	OUTCOME
			MEDICATION PERSCRIBED
NOTES			TREATMENT
			FOLLOW UP

DATE	TIME	DOCTOR	CONTACT
REASON FOR VISIT		QUESTIONS	OUTCOME
			MEDICATION PERSCRIBED
NOTES			TREATMENT
			FOLLOW UP

DATE	TIME	DOCTOR	CONTACT
REASON FOR VISIT		QUESTIONS	OUTCOME
			MEDICATION PERSCRIBED
NOTES			TREATMENT
			FOLLOW UP

DATE	TIME	DOCTOR		CONTACT
REASON FOR VISIT		**QUESTIONS**		**OUTCOME**
				MEDICATION PERSCRIBED
NOTES				**TREATMENT**
				FOLLOW UP

DATE	TIME	DOCTOR		CONTACT
REASON FOR VISIT		**QUESTIONS**		**OUTCOME**
				MEDICATION PERSCRIBED
NOTES				**TREATMENT**
				FOLLOW UP

DATE	TIME	DOCTOR		CONTACT
REASON FOR VISIT		**QUESTIONS**		**OUTCOME**
				MEDICATION PERSCRIBED
NOTES				**TREATMENT**
				FOLLOW UP

DATE	TIME	DOCTOR	CONTACT
REASON FOR VISIT		**QUESTIONS**	**OUTCOME**
			MEDICATION PERSCRIBED
NOTES			**TREATMENT**
			FOLLOW UP

DATE	TIME	DOCTOR	CONTACT
REASON FOR VISIT		**QUESTIONS**	**OUTCOME**
			MEDICATION PERSCRIBED
NOTES			**TREATMENT**
			FOLLOW UP

DATE	TIME	DOCTOR	CONTACT
REASON FOR VISIT		**QUESTIONS**	**OUTCOME**
			MEDICATION PERSCRIBED
NOTES			**TREATMENT**
			FOLLOW UP

DATE	TIME	DOCTOR		CONTACT
REASON FOR VISIT		QUESTIONS		OUTCOME
				MEDICATION PERSCRIBED
NOTES				TREATMENT
				FOLLOW UP

DATE	TIME	DOCTOR		CONTACT
REASON FOR VISIT		QUESTIONS		OUTCOME
				MEDICATION PERSCRIBED
NOTES				TREATMENT
				FOLLOW UP

DATE	TIME	DOCTOR		CONTACT
REASON FOR VISIT		QUESTIONS		OUTCOME
				MEDICATION PERSCRIBED
NOTES				TREATMENT
				FOLLOW UP

DATE	TIME	DOCTOR		CONTACT
REASON FOR VISIT		**QUESTIONS**		**OUTCOME**
				MEDICATION PERSCRIBED
NOTES				**TREATMENT**
				FOLLOW UP

DATE	TIME	DOCTOR		CONTACT
REASON FOR VISIT		**QUESTIONS**		**OUTCOME**
				MEDICATION PERSCRIBED
NOTES				**TREATMENT**
				FOLLOW UP

DATE	TIME	DOCTOR		CONTACT
REASON FOR VISIT		**QUESTIONS**		**OUTCOME**
				MEDICATION PERSCRIBED
NOTES				**TREATMENT**
				FOLLOW UP

DATE	TIME	DOCTOR	CONTACT
REASON FOR VISIT		QUESTIONS	OUTCOME
			MEDICATION PERSCRIBED
NOTES			TREATMENT
			FOLLOW UP

DATE	TIME	DOCTOR	CONTACT
REASON FOR VISIT		QUESTIONS	OUTCOME
			MEDICATION PERSCRIBED
NOTES			TREATMENT
			FOLLOW UP

DATE	TIME	DOCTOR	CONTACT
REASON FOR VISIT		QUESTIONS	OUTCOME
			MEDICATION PERSCRIBED
NOTES			TREATMENT
			FOLLOW UP

DATE	TIME	DOCTOR	CONTACT
REASON FOR VISIT		QUESTIONS	OUTCOME
			MEDICATION PERSCRIBED
NOTES			TREATMENT
			FOLLOW UP

DATE	TIME	DOCTOR	CONTACT
REASON FOR VISIT		QUESTIONS	OUTCOME
			MEDICATION PERSCRIBED
NOTES			TREATMENT
			FOLLOW UP

DATE	TIME	DOCTOR	CONTACT
REASON FOR VISIT		QUESTIONS	OUTCOME
			MEDICATION PERSCRIBED
NOTES			TREATMENT
			FOLLOW UP

DATE	TIME	DOCTOR		CONTACT
REASON FOR VISIT		QUESTIONS		OUTCOME
				MEDICATION PERSCRIBED
NOTES				TREATMENT
				FOLLOW UP

DATE	TIME	DOCTOR		CONTACT
REASON FOR VISIT		QUESTIONS		OUTCOME
				MEDICATION PERSCRIBED
NOTES				TREATMENT
				FOLLOW UP

DATE	TIME	DOCTOR		CONTACT
REASON FOR VISIT		QUESTIONS		OUTCOME
				MEDICATION PERSCRIBED
NOTES				TREATMENT
				FOLLOW UP

DATE	TIME	DOCTOR	CONTACT
REASON FOR VISIT		QUESTIONS	OUTCOME
			MEDICATION PERSCRIBED
NOTES			TREATMENT
			FOLLOW UP

DATE	TIME	DOCTOR	CONTACT
REASON FOR VISIT		QUESTIONS	OUTCOME
			MEDICATION PERSCRIBED
NOTES			TREATMENT
			FOLLOW UP

DATE	TIME	DOCTOR	CONTACT
REASON FOR VISIT		QUESTIONS	OUTCOME
			MEDICATION PERSCRIBED
NOTES			TREATMENT
			FOLLOW UP

DATE	TIME	DOCTOR		CONTACT
REASON FOR VISIT		QUESTIONS		OUTCOME
				MEDICATION PERSCRIBED
NOTES				TREATMENT
				FOLLOW UP

DATE	TIME	DOCTOR		CONTACT
REASON FOR VISIT		QUESTIONS		OUTCOME
				MEDICATION PERSCRIBED
NOTES				TREATMENT
				FOLLOW UP

DATE	TIME	DOCTOR		CONTACT
REASON FOR VISIT		QUESTIONS		OUTCOME
				MEDICATION PERSCRIBED
NOTES				TREATMENT
				FOLLOW UP

DATE	TIME	DOCTOR		CONTACT
REASON FOR VISIT		QUESTIONS		OUTCOME
				MEDICATION PERSCRIBED
NOTES				TREATMENT
				FOLLOW UP

DATE	TIME	DOCTOR		CONTACT
REASON FOR VISIT		QUESTIONS		OUTCOME
				MEDICATION PERSCRIBED
NOTES				TREATMENT
				FOLLOW UP

DATE	TIME	DOCTOR		CONTACT
REASON FOR VISIT		QUESTIONS		OUTCOME
				MEDICATION PERSCRIBED
NOTES				TREATMENT
				FOLLOW UP

DATE	TIME	DOCTOR		CONTACT	
REASON FOR VISIT		QUESTIONS		OUTCOME	
				MEDICATION PERSCRIBED	
NOTES				TREATMENT	
				FOLLOW UP	

DATE	TIME	DOCTOR		CONTACT	
REASON FOR VISIT		QUESTIONS		OUTCOME	
				MEDICATION PERSCRIBED	
NOTES				TREATMENT	
				FOLLOW UP	

DATE	TIME	DOCTOR		CONTACT	
REASON FOR VISIT		QUESTIONS		OUTCOME	
				MEDICATION PERSCRIBED	
NOTES				TREATMENT	
				FOLLOW UP	

DATE	TIME	DOCTOR	CONTACT
REASON FOR VISIT		QUESTIONS	OUTCOME
			MEDICATION PERSCRIBED
NOTES			TREATMENT
			FOLLOW UP

DATE	TIME	DOCTOR	CONTACT
REASON FOR VISIT		QUESTIONS	OUTCOME
			MEDICATION PERSCRIBED
NOTES			TREATMENT
			FOLLOW UP

DATE	TIME	DOCTOR	CONTACT
REASON FOR VISIT		QUESTIONS	OUTCOME
			MEDICATION PERSCRIBED
NOTES			TREATMENT
			FOLLOW UP

DATE	TIME	DOCTOR		CONTACT
REASON FOR VISIT		QUESTIONS		OUTCOME
				MEDICATION PERSCRIBED
NOTES				TREATMENT
				FOLLOW UP

DATE	TIME	DOCTOR		CONTACT
REASON FOR VISIT		QUESTIONS		OUTCOME
				MEDICATION PERSCRIBED
NOTES				TREATMENT
				FOLLOW UP

DATE	TIME	DOCTOR		CONTACT
REASON FOR VISIT		QUESTIONS		OUTCOME
				MEDICATION PERSCRIBED
NOTES				TREATMENT
				FOLLOW UP

DATE	TIME	DOCTOR		CONTACT
REASON FOR VISIT		QUESTIONS		OUTCOME
				MEDICATION PERSCRIBED
NOTES				TREATMENT
				FOLLOW UP

DATE	TIME	DOCTOR		CONTACT
REASON FOR VISIT		QUESTIONS		OUTCOME
				MEDICATION PERSCRIBED
NOTES				TREATMENT
				FOLLOW UP

DATE	TIME	DOCTOR		CONTACT
REASON FOR VISIT		QUESTIONS		OUTCOME
				MEDICATION PERSCRIBED
NOTES				TREATMENT
				FOLLOW UP

DATE	TIME	DOCTOR		CONTACT
REASON FOR VISIT		**QUESTIONS**		**OUTCOME**
				MEDICATION PERSCRIBED
NOTES				**TREATMENT**
				FOLLOW UP

DATE	TIME	DOCTOR		CONTACT
REASON FOR VISIT		**QUESTIONS**		**OUTCOME**
				MEDICATION PERSCRIBED
NOTES				**TREATMENT**
				FOLLOW UP

DATE	TIME	DOCTOR		CONTACT
REASON FOR VISIT		**QUESTIONS**		**OUTCOME**
				MEDICATION PERSCRIBED
NOTES				**TREATMENT**
				FOLLOW UP

DATE	TIME	DOCTOR	CONTACT
REASON FOR VISIT		QUESTIONS	OUTCOME
			MEDICATION PERSCRIBED
NOTES			TREATMENT
			FOLLOW UP

DATE	TIME	DOCTOR	CONTACT
REASON FOR VISIT		QUESTIONS	OUTCOME
			MEDICATION PERSCRIBED
NOTES			TREATMENT
			FOLLOW UP

DATE	TIME	DOCTOR	CONTACT
REASON FOR VISIT		QUESTIONS	OUTCOME
			MEDICATION PERSCRIBED
NOTES			TREATMENT
			FOLLOW UP

DATE	TIME	DOCTOR		CONTACT
REASON FOR VISIT		QUESTIONS		OUTCOME
				MEDICATION PERSCRIBED
NOTES				TREATMENT
				FOLLOW UP

DATE	TIME	DOCTOR		CONTACT
REASON FOR VISIT		QUESTIONS		OUTCOME
				MEDICATION PERSCRIBED
NOTES				TREATMENT
				FOLLOW UP

DATE	TIME	DOCTOR		CONTACT
REASON FOR VISIT		QUESTIONS		OUTCOME
				MEDICATION PERSCRIBED
NOTES				TREATMENT
				FOLLOW UP

DATE	TIME	DOCTOR		CONTACT
REASON FOR VISIT		QUESTIONS		OUTCOME
				MEDICATION PERSCRIBED
NOTES				TREATMENT
				FOLLOW UP

DATE	TIME	DOCTOR		CONTACT
REASON FOR VISIT		QUESTIONS		OUTCOME
				MEDICATION PERSCRIBED
NOTES				TREATMENT
				FOLLOW UP

DATE	TIME	DOCTOR		CONTACT
REASON FOR VISIT		QUESTIONS		OUTCOME
				MEDICATION PERSCRIBED
NOTES				TREATMENT
				FOLLOW UP

DATE	TIME	DOCTOR		CONTACT
REASON FOR VISIT		QUESTIONS		OUTCOME
				MEDICATION PERSCRIBED
NOTES				TREATMENT
				FOLLOW UP

DATE	TIME	DOCTOR		CONTACT
REASON FOR VISIT		QUESTIONS		OUTCOME
				MEDICATION PERSCRIBED
NOTES				TREATMENT
				FOLLOW UP

DATE	TIME	DOCTOR		CONTACT
REASON FOR VISIT		QUESTIONS		OUTCOME
				MEDICATION PERSCRIBED
NOTES				TREATMENT
				FOLLOW UP

DATE	TIME	DOCTOR		CONTACT
REASON FOR VISIT		QUESTIONS		OUTCOME
				MEDICATION PERSCRIBED
NOTES				TREATMENT
				FOLLOW UP

DATE	TIME	DOCTOR		CONTACT
REASON FOR VISIT		QUESTIONS		OUTCOME
				MEDICATION PERSCRIBED
NOTES				TREATMENT
				FOLLOW UP

DATE	TIME	DOCTOR		CONTACT
REASON FOR VISIT		QUESTIONS		OUTCOME
				MEDICATION PERSCRIBED
NOTES				TREATMENT
				FOLLOW UP

DATE	TIME	DOCTOR		CONTACT
REASON FOR VISIT		QUESTIONS		OUTCOME
				MEDICATION PERSCRIBED
NOTES				TREATMENT
				FOLLOW UP

DATE	TIME	DOCTOR		CONTACT
REASON FOR VISIT		QUESTIONS		OUTCOME
				MEDICATION PERSCRIBED
NOTES				TREATMENT
				FOLLOW UP

DATE	TIME	DOCTOR		CONTACT
REASON FOR VISIT		QUESTIONS		OUTCOME
				MEDICATION PERSCRIBED
NOTES				TREATMENT
				FOLLOW UP

DATE	TIME	DOCTOR		CONTACT
REASON FOR VISIT		QUESTIONS		OUTCOME
				MEDICATION PERSCRIBED
NOTES				TREATMENT
				FOLLOW UP

DATE	TIME	DOCTOR		CONTACT
REASON FOR VISIT		QUESTIONS		OUTCOME
				MEDICATION PERSCRIBED
NOTES				TREATMENT
				FOLLOW UP

DATE	TIME	DOCTOR		CONTACT
REASON FOR VISIT		QUESTIONS		OUTCOME
				MEDICATION PERSCRIBED
NOTES				TREATMENT
				FOLLOW UP

DATE	TIME	DOCTOR		CONTACT
REASON FOR VISIT		QUESTIONS		OUTCOME
				MEDICATION PERSCRIBED
NOTES				TREATMENT
				FOLLOW UP

DATE	TIME	DOCTOR		CONTACT
REASON FOR VISIT		QUESTIONS		OUTCOME
				MEDICATION PERSCRIBED
NOTES				TREATMENT
				FOLLOW UP

DATE	TIME	DOCTOR		CONTACT
REASON FOR VISIT		QUESTIONS		OUTCOME
				MEDICATION PERSCRIBED
NOTES				TREATMENT
				FOLLOW UP

DATE	TIME	DOCTOR	CONTACT

REASON FOR VISIT	QUESTIONS	OUTCOME
		MEDICATION PERSCRIBED

NOTES	TREATMENT
	FOLLOW UP

DATE	TIME	DOCTOR	CONTACT

REASON FOR VISIT	QUESTIONS	OUTCOME
		MEDICATION PERSCRIBED

NOTES	TREATMENT
	FOLLOW UP

DATE	TIME	DOCTOR	CONTACT

REASON FOR VISIT	QUESTIONS	OUTCOME
		MEDICATION PERSCRIBED

NOTES	TREATMENT
	FOLLOW UP

DATE	TIME	DOCTOR		CONTACT
REASON FOR VISIT		QUESTIONS		OUTCOME
				MEDICATION PERSCRIBED
NOTES				TREATMENT
				FOLLOW UP

DATE	TIME	DOCTOR		CONTACT
REASON FOR VISIT		QUESTIONS		OUTCOME
				MEDICATION PERSCRIBED
NOTES				TREATMENT
				FOLLOW UP

DATE	TIME	DOCTOR		CONTACT
REASON FOR VISIT		QUESTIONS		OUTCOME
				MEDICATION PERSCRIBED
NOTES				TREATMENT
				FOLLOW UP

DATE	TIME	DOCTOR		CONTACT
REASON FOR VISIT		QUESTIONS		OUTCOME
				MEDICATION PERSCRIBED
NOTES				TREATMENT
				FOLLOW UP

DATE	TIME	DOCTOR		CONTACT
REASON FOR VISIT		QUESTIONS		OUTCOME
				MEDICATION PERSCRIBED
NOTES				TREATMENT
				FOLLOW UP

DATE	TIME	DOCTOR		CONTACT
REASON FOR VISIT		QUESTIONS		OUTCOME
				MEDICATION PERSCRIBED
NOTES				TREATMENT
				FOLLOW UP

DATE	TIME	DOCTOR		CONTACT
REASON FOR VISIT		QUESTIONS		OUTCOME
				MEDICATION PERSCRIBED
NOTES				TREATMENT
				FOLLOW UP

DATE	TIME	DOCTOR		CONTACT
REASON FOR VISIT		QUESTIONS		OUTCOME
				MEDICATION PERSCRIBED
NOTES				TREATMENT
				FOLLOW UP

DATE	TIME	DOCTOR		CONTACT
REASON FOR VISIT		QUESTIONS		OUTCOME
				MEDICATION PERSCRIBED
NOTES				TREATMENT
				FOLLOW UP

DATE	TIME	DOCTOR		CONTACT
REASON FOR VISIT		QUESTIONS		OUTCOME
				MEDICATION PERSCRIBED
NOTES				TREATMENT
				FOLLOW UP

DATE	TIME	DOCTOR		CONTACT
REASON FOR VISIT		QUESTIONS		OUTCOME
				MEDICATION PERSCRIBED
NOTES				TREATMENT
				FOLLOW UP

DATE	TIME	DOCTOR		CONTACT
REASON FOR VISIT		QUESTIONS		OUTCOME
				MEDICATION PERSCRIBED
NOTES				TREATMENT
				FOLLOW UP

DATE	TIME	DOCTOR	CONTACT
REASON FOR VISIT		QUESTIONS	OUTCOME
			MEDICATION PERSCRIBED
NOTES			TREATMENT
			FOLLOW UP

DATE	TIME	DOCTOR	CONTACT
REASON FOR VISIT		QUESTIONS	OUTCOME
			MEDICATION PERSCRIBED
NOTES			TREATMENT
			FOLLOW UP

DATE	TIME	DOCTOR	CONTACT
REASON FOR VISIT		QUESTIONS	OUTCOME
			MEDICATION PERSCRIBED
NOTES			TREATMENT
			FOLLOW UP

DATE	TIME	DOCTOR		CONTACT
REASON FOR VISIT		QUESTIONS		OUTCOME
				MEDICATION PERSCRIBED
NOTES				TREATMENT
				FOLLOW UP

DATE	TIME	DOCTOR		CONTACT
REASON FOR VISIT		QUESTIONS		OUTCOME
				MEDICATION PERSCRIBED
NOTES				TREATMENT
				FOLLOW UP

DATE	TIME	DOCTOR		CONTACT
REASON FOR VISIT		QUESTIONS		OUTCOME
				MEDICATION PERSCRIBED
NOTES				TREATMENT
				FOLLOW UP

DATE	TIME	DOCTOR		CONTACT	
REASON FOR VISIT		QUESTIONS		OUTCOME	
				MEDICATION PERSCRIBED	
NOTES				TREATMENT	
				FOLLOW UP	

DATE	TIME	DOCTOR		CONTACT	
REASON FOR VISIT		QUESTIONS		OUTCOME	
				MEDICATION PERSCRIBED	
NOTES				TREATMENT	
				FOLLOW UP	

DATE	TIME	DOCTOR		CONTACT	
REASON FOR VISIT		QUESTIONS		OUTCOME	
				MEDICATION PERSCRIBED	
NOTES				TREATMENT	
				FOLLOW UP	

DATE	TIME	DOCTOR		CONTACT
REASON FOR VISIT		QUESTIONS		OUTCOME
				MEDICATION PERSCRIBED
NOTES				TREATMENT
				FOLLOW UP

DATE	TIME	DOCTOR		CONTACT
REASON FOR VISIT		QUESTIONS		OUTCOME
				MEDICATION PERSCRIBED
NOTES				TREATMENT
				FOLLOW UP

DATE	TIME	DOCTOR		CONTACT
REASON FOR VISIT		QUESTIONS		OUTCOME
				MEDICATION PERSCRIBED
NOTES				TREATMENT
				FOLLOW UP

DATE	TIME	DOCTOR		CONTACT
REASON FOR VISIT		QUESTIONS		OUTCOME
				MEDICATION PERSCRIBED
NOTES				TREATMENT
				FOLLOW UP

DATE	TIME	DOCTOR		CONTACT
REASON FOR VISIT		QUESTIONS		OUTCOME
				MEDICATION PERSCRIBED
NOTES				TREATMENT
				FOLLOW UP

DATE	TIME	DOCTOR		CONTACT
REASON FOR VISIT		QUESTIONS		OUTCOME
				MEDICATION PERSCRIBED
NOTES				TREATMENT
				FOLLOW UP

DATE	TIME	DOCTOR		CONTACT
REASON FOR VISIT		QUESTIONS		OUTCOME
				MEDICATION PERSCRIBED
NOTES				TREATMENT
				FOLLOW UP

DATE	TIME	DOCTOR		CONTACT
REASON FOR VISIT		QUESTIONS		OUTCOME
				MEDICATION PERSCRIBED
NOTES				TREATMENT
				FOLLOW UP

DATE	TIME	DOCTOR		CONTACT
REASON FOR VISIT		QUESTIONS		OUTCOME
				MEDICATION PERSCRIBED
NOTES				TREATMENT
				FOLLOW UP

DATE	TIME	DOCTOR		CONTACT
REASON FOR VISIT		**QUESTIONS**		**OUTCOME**
				MEDICATION PERSCRIBED
NOTES				**TREATMENT**
				FOLLOW UP

DATE	TIME	DOCTOR		CONTACT
REASON FOR VISIT		**QUESTIONS**		**OUTCOME**
				MEDICATION PERSCRIBED
NOTES				**TREATMENT**
				FOLLOW UP

DATE	TIME	DOCTOR		CONTACT
REASON FOR VISIT		**QUESTIONS**		**OUTCOME**
				MEDICATION PERSCRIBED
NOTES				**TREATMENT**
				FOLLOW UP

DATE	TIME	DOCTOR		CONTACT
REASON FOR VISIT		QUESTIONS		OUTCOME
				MEDICATION PERSCRIBED
NOTES				TREATMENT
				FOLLOW UP

DATE	TIME	DOCTOR		CONTACT
REASON FOR VISIT		QUESTIONS		OUTCOME
				MEDICATION PERSCRIBED
NOTES				TREATMENT
				FOLLOW UP

DATE	TIME	DOCTOR		CONTACT
REASON FOR VISIT		QUESTIONS		OUTCOME
				MEDICATION PERSCRIBED
NOTES				TREATMENT
				FOLLOW UP

DATE	TIME	DOCTOR		CONTACT
REASON FOR VISIT		**QUESTIONS**		**OUTCOME**
				MEDICATION PERSCRIBED
NOTES				**TREATMENT**
				FOLLOW UP

DATE	TIME	DOCTOR		CONTACT
REASON FOR VISIT		**QUESTIONS**		**OUTCOME**
				MEDICATION PERSCRIBED
NOTES				**TREATMENT**
				FOLLOW UP

DATE	TIME	DOCTOR		CONTACT
REASON FOR VISIT		**QUESTIONS**		**OUTCOME**
				MEDICATION PERSCRIBED
NOTES				**TREATMENT**
				FOLLOW UP

DATE	TIME	DOCTOR		CONTACT
REASON FOR VISIT		QUESTIONS		OUTCOME
				MEDICATION PERSCRIBED
NOTES				TREATMENT
				FOLLOW UP

DATE	TIME	DOCTOR		CONTACT
REASON FOR VISIT		QUESTIONS		OUTCOME
				MEDICATION PERSCRIBED
NOTES				TREATMENT
				FOLLOW UP

DATE	TIME	DOCTOR		CONTACT
REASON FOR VISIT		QUESTIONS		OUTCOME
				MEDICATION PERSCRIBED
NOTES				TREATMENT
				FOLLOW UP

DATE	TIME	DOCTOR		CONTACT
REASON FOR VISIT		QUESTIONS		OUTCOME
				MEDICATION PERSCRIBED
NOTES				TREATMENT
				FOLLOW UP

DATE	TIME	DOCTOR		CONTACT
REASON FOR VISIT		QUESTIONS		OUTCOME
				MEDICATION PERSCRIBED
NOTES				TREATMENT
				FOLLOW UP

DATE	TIME	DOCTOR		CONTACT
REASON FOR VISIT		QUESTIONS		OUTCOME
				MEDICATION PERSCRIBED
NOTES				TREATMENT
				FOLLOW UP

DATE	TIME	DOCTOR	CONTACT

REASON FOR VISIT	QUESTIONS	OUTCOME
		MEDICATION PERSCRIBED

NOTES	TREATMENT
	FOLLOW UP

DATE	TIME	DOCTOR	CONTACT

REASON FOR VISIT	QUESTIONS	OUTCOME
		MEDICATION PERSCRIBED

NOTES	TREATMENT
	FOLLOW UP

DATE	TIME	DOCTOR	CONTACT

REASON FOR VISIT	QUESTIONS	OUTCOME
		MEDICATION PERSCRIBED

NOTES	TREATMENT
	FOLLOW UP

DATE	TIME	DOCTOR		CONTACT
REASON FOR VISIT		QUESTIONS		OUTCOME
				MEDICATION PERSCRIBED
NOTES				TREATMENT
				FOLLOW UP

DATE	TIME	DOCTOR		CONTACT
REASON FOR VISIT		QUESTIONS		OUTCOME
				MEDICATION PERSCRIBED
NOTES				TREATMENT
				FOLLOW UP

DATE	TIME	DOCTOR		CONTACT
REASON FOR VISIT		QUESTIONS		OUTCOME
				MEDICATION PERSCRIBED
NOTES				TREATMENT
				FOLLOW UP

DATE	TIME	DOCTOR		CONTACT
REASON FOR VISIT		QUESTIONS		OUTCOME
				MEDICATION PERSCRIBED
NOTES				TREATMENT
				FOLLOW UP

DATE	TIME	DOCTOR		CONTACT
REASON FOR VISIT		QUESTIONS		OUTCOME
				MEDICATION PERSCRIBED
NOTES				TREATMENT
				FOLLOW UP

DATE	TIME	DOCTOR		CONTACT
REASON FOR VISIT		QUESTIONS		OUTCOME
				MEDICATION PERSCRIBED
NOTES				TREATMENT
				FOLLOW UP

DATE	TIME	DOCTOR	CONTACT
REASON FOR VISIT		QUESTIONS	OUTCOME
			MEDICATION PERSCRIBED
NOTES			TREATMENT
			FOLLOW UP

DATE	TIME	DOCTOR	CONTACT
REASON FOR VISIT		QUESTIONS	OUTCOME
			MEDICATION PERSCRIBED
NOTES			TREATMENT
			FOLLOW UP

DATE	TIME	DOCTOR	CONTACT
REASON FOR VISIT		QUESTIONS	OUTCOME
			MEDICATION PERSCRIBED
NOTES			TREATMENT
			FOLLOW UP

DATE	TIME	DOCTOR	CONTACT
REASON FOR VISIT		QUESTIONS	OUTCOME
			MEDICATION PERSCRIBED
NOTES			TREATMENT
			FOLLOW UP

DATE	TIME	DOCTOR	CONTACT
REASON FOR VISIT		QUESTIONS	OUTCOME
			MEDICATION PERSCRIBED
NOTES			TREATMENT
			FOLLOW UP

DATE	TIME	DOCTOR	CONTACT
REASON FOR VISIT		QUESTIONS	OUTCOME
			MEDICATION PERSCRIBED
NOTES			TREATMENT
			FOLLOW UP

DATE	TIME	DOCTOR		CONTACT
REASON FOR VISIT		QUESTIONS		OUTCOME
				MEDICATION PERSCRIBED
NOTES				TREATMENT
				FOLLOW UP

DATE	TIME	DOCTOR		CONTACT
REASON FOR VISIT		QUESTIONS		OUTCOME
				MEDICATION PERSCRIBED
NOTES				TREATMENT
				FOLLOW UP

DATE	TIME	DOCTOR		CONTACT
REASON FOR VISIT		QUESTIONS		OUTCOME
				MEDICATION PERSCRIBED
NOTES				TREATMENT
				FOLLOW UP

DATE	TIME	DOCTOR	CONTACT
REASON FOR VISIT		QUESTIONS	OUTCOME
			MEDICATION PERSCRIBED
NOTES			TREATMENT
			FOLLOW UP

DATE	TIME	DOCTOR	CONTACT
REASON FOR VISIT		QUESTIONS	OUTCOME
			MEDICATION PERSCRIBED
NOTES			TREATMENT
			FOLLOW UP

DATE	TIME	DOCTOR	CONTACT
REASON FOR VISIT		QUESTIONS	OUTCOME
			MEDICATION PERSCRIBED
NOTES			TREATMENT
			FOLLOW UP

DATE	TIME	DOCTOR		CONTACT
REASON FOR VISIT		QUESTIONS		OUTCOME
				MEDICATION PERSCRIBED
NOTES				TREATMENT
				FOLLOW UP

DATE	TIME	DOCTOR		CONTACT
REASON FOR VISIT		QUESTIONS		OUTCOME
				MEDICATION PERSCRIBED
NOTES				TREATMENT
				FOLLOW UP

DATE	TIME	DOCTOR		CONTACT
REASON FOR VISIT		QUESTIONS		OUTCOME
				MEDICATION PERSCRIBED
NOTES				TREATMENT
				FOLLOW UP

DATE	TIME	DOCTOR		CONTACT
REASON FOR VISIT		QUESTIONS		OUTCOME
				MEDICATION PERSCRIBED
NOTES				TREATMENT
				FOLLOW UP

DATE	TIME	DOCTOR		CONTACT
REASON FOR VISIT		QUESTIONS		OUTCOME
				MEDICATION PERSCRIBED
NOTES				TREATMENT
				FOLLOW UP

DATE	TIME	DOCTOR		CONTACT
REASON FOR VISIT		QUESTIONS		OUTCOME
				MEDICATION PERSCRIBED
NOTES				TREATMENT
				FOLLOW UP

DATE	TIME	DOCTOR	CONTACT
REASON FOR VISIT		QUESTIONS	OUTCOME
			MEDICATION PERSCRIBED
NOTES			TREATMENT
			FOLLOW UP

DATE	TIME	DOCTOR	CONTACT
REASON FOR VISIT		QUESTIONS	OUTCOME
			MEDICATION PERSCRIBED
NOTES			TREATMENT
			FOLLOW UP

DATE	TIME	DOCTOR	CONTACT
REASON FOR VISIT		QUESTIONS	OUTCOME
			MEDICATION PERSCRIBED
NOTES			TREATMENT
			FOLLOW UP

DATE	TIME	DOCTOR		CONTACT
REASON FOR VISIT		QUESTIONS		OUTCOME
				MEDICATION PERSCRIBED
NOTES				TREATMENT
				FOLLOW UP

DATE	TIME	DOCTOR		CONTACT
REASON FOR VISIT		QUESTIONS		OUTCOME
				MEDICATION PERSCRIBED
NOTES				TREATMENT
				FOLLOW UP

DATE	TIME	DOCTOR		CONTACT
REASON FOR VISIT		QUESTIONS		OUTCOME
				MEDICATION PERSCRIBED
NOTES				TREATMENT
				FOLLOW UP

DATE	TIME	DOCTOR	CONTACT
REASON FOR VISIT		QUESTIONS	OUTCOME
			MEDICATION PERSCRIBED
NOTES			TREATMENT
			FOLLOW UP

DATE	TIME	DOCTOR	CONTACT
REASON FOR VISIT		QUESTIONS	OUTCOME
			MEDICATION PERSCRIBED
NOTES			TREATMENT
			FOLLOW UP

DATE	TIME	DOCTOR	CONTACT
REASON FOR VISIT		QUESTIONS	OUTCOME
			MEDICATION PERSCRIBED
NOTES			TREATMENT
			FOLLOW UP

DATE	TIME	DOCTOR		CONTACT
REASON FOR VISIT		QUESTIONS		OUTCOME
				MEDICATION PERSCRIBED
NOTES				TREATMENT
				FOLLOW UP

DATE	TIME	DOCTOR		CONTACT
REASON FOR VISIT		QUESTIONS		OUTCOME
				MEDICATION PERSCRIBED
NOTES				TREATMENT
				FOLLOW UP

DATE	TIME	DOCTOR		CONTACT
REASON FOR VISIT		QUESTIONS		OUTCOME
				MEDICATION PERSCRIBED
NOTES				TREATMENT
				FOLLOW UP

DATE	TIME	DOCTOR	CONTACT

REASON FOR VISIT	QUESTIONS	OUTCOME
		MEDICATION PERSCRIBED
NOTES		TREATMENT
		FOLLOW UP

DATE	TIME	DOCTOR	CONTACT

REASON FOR VISIT	QUESTIONS	OUTCOME
		MEDICATION PERSCRIBED
NOTES		TREATMENT
		FOLLOW UP

DATE	TIME	DOCTOR	CONTACT

REASON FOR VISIT	QUESTIONS	OUTCOME
		MEDICATION PERSCRIBED
NOTES		TREATMENT
		FOLLOW UP

DATE	TIME	DOCTOR		CONTACT
REASON FOR VISIT		QUESTIONS		OUTCOME
				MEDICATION PERSCRIBED
NOTES				TREATMENT
				FOLLOW UP

DATE	TIME	DOCTOR		CONTACT
REASON FOR VISIT		QUESTIONS		OUTCOME
				MEDICATION PERSCRIBED
NOTES				TREATMENT
				FOLLOW UP

DATE	TIME	DOCTOR		CONTACT
REASON FOR VISIT		QUESTIONS		OUTCOME
				MEDICATION PERSCRIBED
NOTES				TREATMENT
				FOLLOW UP

DATE	TIME	DOCTOR		CONTACT
REASON FOR VISIT		QUESTIONS		OUTCOME
				MEDICATION PERSCRIBED
NOTES				TREATMENT
				FOLLOW UP

DATE	TIME	DOCTOR		CONTACT
REASON FOR VISIT		QUESTIONS		OUTCOME
				MEDICATION PERSCRIBED
NOTES				TREATMENT
				FOLLOW UP

DATE	TIME	DOCTOR		CONTACT
REASON FOR VISIT		QUESTIONS		OUTCOME
				MEDICATION PERSCRIBED
NOTES				TREATMENT
				FOLLOW UP

DATE	TIME	DOCTOR	CONTACT
REASON FOR VISIT		**QUESTIONS**	**OUTCOME**
			MEDICATION PERSCRIBED
NOTES			**TREATMENT**
			FOLLOW UP

DATE	TIME	DOCTOR	CONTACT
REASON FOR VISIT		**QUESTIONS**	**OUTCOME**
			MEDICATION PERSCRIBED
NOTES			**TREATMENT**
			FOLLOW UP

DATE	TIME	DOCTOR	CONTACT
REASON FOR VISIT		**QUESTIONS**	**OUTCOME**
			MEDICATION PERSCRIBED
NOTES			**TREATMENT**
			FOLLOW UP

DATE	TIME	DOCTOR		CONTACT
REASON FOR VISIT		QUESTIONS		OUTCOME
				MEDICATION PERSCRIBED
NOTES				TREATMENT
				FOLLOW UP

DATE	TIME	DOCTOR		CONTACT
REASON FOR VISIT		QUESTIONS		OUTCOME
				MEDICATION PERSCRIBED
NOTES				TREATMENT
				FOLLOW UP

DATE	TIME	DOCTOR		CONTACT
REASON FOR VISIT		QUESTIONS		OUTCOME
				MEDICATION PERSCRIBED
NOTES				TREATMENT
				FOLLOW UP

DATE	TIME	DOCTOR	CONTACT
REASON FOR VISIT		QUESTIONS	OUTCOME
			MEDICATION PERSCRIBED
NOTES			TREATMENT
			FOLLOW UP

DATE	TIME	DOCTOR	CONTACT
REASON FOR VISIT		QUESTIONS	OUTCOME
			MEDICATION PERSCRIBED
NOTES			TREATMENT
			FOLLOW UP

DATE	TIME	DOCTOR	CONTACT
REASON FOR VISIT		QUESTIONS	OUTCOME
			MEDICATION PERSCRIBED
NOTES			TREATMENT
			FOLLOW UP

DATE	TIME	DOCTOR		CONTACT
REASON FOR VISIT		**QUESTIONS**		**OUTCOME**
				MEDICATION PERSCRIBED
NOTES				**TREATMENT**
				FOLLOW UP

DATE	TIME	DOCTOR		CONTACT
REASON FOR VISIT		**QUESTIONS**		**OUTCOME**
				MEDICATION PERSCRIBED
NOTES				**TREATMENT**
				FOLLOW UP

DATE	TIME	DOCTOR		CONTACT
REASON FOR VISIT		**QUESTIONS**		**OUTCOME**
				MEDICATION PERSCRIBED
NOTES				**TREATMENT**
				FOLLOW UP

DATE	TIME	DOCTOR		CONTACT
REASON FOR VISIT		QUESTIONS		OUTCOME
				MEDICATION PERSCRIBED
NOTES				TREATMENT
				FOLLOW UP

DATE	TIME	DOCTOR		CONTACT
REASON FOR VISIT		QUESTIONS		OUTCOME
				MEDICATION PERSCRIBED
NOTES				TREATMENT
				FOLLOW UP

DATE	TIME	DOCTOR		CONTACT
REASON FOR VISIT		QUESTIONS		OUTCOME
				MEDICATION PERSCRIBED
NOTES				TREATMENT
				FOLLOW UP

DATE	TIME	DOCTOR		CONTACT
REASON FOR VISIT		QUESTIONS		OUTCOME
				MEDICATION PERSCRIBED
NOTES				TREATMENT
				FOLLOW UP

DATE	TIME	DOCTOR		CONTACT
REASON FOR VISIT		QUESTIONS		OUTCOME
				MEDICATION PERSCRIBED
NOTES				TREATMENT
				FOLLOW UP

DATE	TIME	DOCTOR		CONTACT
REASON FOR VISIT		QUESTIONS		OUTCOME
				MEDICATION PERSCRIBED
NOTES				TREATMENT
				FOLLOW UP

DATE	TIME	DOCTOR		CONTACT
REASON FOR VISIT		QUESTIONS		OUTCOME
				MEDICATION PERSCRIBED
NOTES				TREATMENT
				FOLLOW UP

DATE	TIME	DOCTOR		CONTACT
REASON FOR VISIT		QUESTIONS		OUTCOME
				MEDICATION PERSCRIBED
NOTES				TREATMENT
				FOLLOW UP

DATE	TIME	DOCTOR		CONTACT
REASON FOR VISIT		QUESTIONS		OUTCOME
				MEDICATION PERSCRIBED
NOTES				TREATMENT
				FOLLOW UP

DATE	TIME	DOCTOR		CONTACT
REASON FOR VISIT		QUESTIONS		OUTCOME
				MEDICATION PERSCRIBED
NOTES				TREATMENT
				FOLLOW UP

DATE	TIME	DOCTOR		CONTACT
REASON FOR VISIT		QUESTIONS		OUTCOME
				MEDICATION PERSCRIBED
NOTES				TREATMENT
				FOLLOW UP

DATE	TIME	DOCTOR		CONTACT
REASON FOR VISIT		QUESTIONS		OUTCOME
				MEDICATION PERSCRIBED
NOTES				TREATMENT
				FOLLOW UP

DATE	TIME	DOCTOR		CONTACT
REASON FOR VISIT		QUESTIONS		OUTCOME
				MEDICATION PERSCRIBED
NOTES				TREATMENT
				FOLLOW UP

DATE	TIME	DOCTOR		CONTACT
REASON FOR VISIT		QUESTIONS		OUTCOME
				MEDICATION PERSCRIBED
NOTES				TREATMENT
				FOLLOW UP

DATE	TIME	DOCTOR		CONTACT
REASON FOR VISIT		QUESTIONS		OUTCOME
				MEDICATION PERSCRIBED
NOTES				TREATMENT
				FOLLOW UP

DATE	TIME	DOCTOR		CONTACT
REASON FOR VISIT		QUESTIONS		OUTCOME
				MEDICATION PERSCRIBED
NOTES				TREATMENT
				FOLLOW UP

DATE	TIME	DOCTOR		CONTACT
REASON FOR VISIT		QUESTIONS		OUTCOME
				MEDICATION PERSCRIBED
NOTES				TREATMENT
				FOLLOW UP

DATE	TIME	DOCTOR		CONTACT
REASON FOR VISIT		QUESTIONS		OUTCOME
				MEDICATION PERSCRIBED
NOTES				TREATMENT
				FOLLOW UP

DATE	TIME	DOCTOR	CONTACT
REASON FOR VISIT		QUESTIONS	OUTCOME
			MEDICATION PERSCRIBED
NOTES			TREATMENT
			FOLLOW UP

DATE	TIME	DOCTOR	CONTACT
REASON FOR VISIT		QUESTIONS	OUTCOME
			MEDICATION PERSCRIBED
NOTES			TREATMENT
			FOLLOW UP

DATE	TIME	DOCTOR	CONTACT
REASON FOR VISIT		QUESTIONS	OUTCOME
			MEDICATION PERSCRIBED
NOTES			TREATMENT
			FOLLOW UP

DATE	TIME	DOCTOR	CONTACT
REASON FOR VISIT		QUESTIONS	OUTCOME
			MEDICATION PERSCRIBED
NOTES			TREATMENT
			FOLLOW UP

DATE	TIME	DOCTOR	CONTACT
REASON FOR VISIT		QUESTIONS	OUTCOME
			MEDICATION PERSCRIBED
NOTES			TREATMENT
			FOLLOW UP

DATE	TIME	DOCTOR	CONTACT
REASON FOR VISIT		QUESTIONS	OUTCOME
			MEDICATION PERSCRIBED
NOTES			TREATMENT
			FOLLOW UP

DATE	TIME	DOCTOR	CONTACT
REASON FOR VISIT		QUESTIONS	OUTCOME
			MEDICATION PERSCRIBED
NOTES			TREATMENT
			FOLLOW UP

DATE	TIME	DOCTOR	CONTACT
REASON FOR VISIT		QUESTIONS	OUTCOME
			MEDICATION PERSCRIBED
NOTES			TREATMENT
			FOLLOW UP

DATE	TIME	DOCTOR	CONTACT
REASON FOR VISIT		QUESTIONS	OUTCOME
			MEDICATION PERSCRIBED
NOTES			TREATMENT
			FOLLOW UP

DATE	TIME	DOCTOR		CONTACT
REASON FOR VISIT		QUESTIONS		OUTCOME
				MEDICATION PERSCRIBED
NOTES				TREATMENT
				FOLLOW UP

DATE	TIME	DOCTOR		CONTACT
REASON FOR VISIT		QUESTIONS		OUTCOME
				MEDICATION PERSCRIBED
NOTES				TREATMENT
				FOLLOW UP

DATE	TIME	DOCTOR		CONTACT
REASON FOR VISIT		QUESTIONS		OUTCOME
				MEDICATION PERSCRIBED
NOTES				TREATMENT
				FOLLOW UP

DATE	TIME	DOCTOR		CONTACT
REASON FOR VISIT		QUESTIONS		OUTCOME
				MEDICATION PERSCRIBED
NOTES				TREATMENT
				FOLLOW UP

DATE	TIME	DOCTOR		CONTACT
REASON FOR VISIT		QUESTIONS		OUTCOME
				MEDICATION PERSCRIBED
NOTES				TREATMENT
				FOLLOW UP

DATE	TIME	DOCTOR		CONTACT
REASON FOR VISIT		QUESTIONS		OUTCOME
				MEDICATION PERSCRIBED
NOTES				TREATMENT
				FOLLOW UP

DATE	TIME	DOCTOR	CONTACT
REASON FOR VISIT		QUESTIONS	OUTCOME
			MEDICATION PERSCRIBED
NOTES			TREATMENT
			FOLLOW UP

DATE	TIME	DOCTOR	CONTACT
REASON FOR VISIT		QUESTIONS	OUTCOME
			MEDICATION PERSCRIBED
NOTES			TREATMENT
			FOLLOW UP

DATE	TIME	DOCTOR	CONTACT
REASON FOR VISIT		QUESTIONS	OUTCOME
			MEDICATION PERSCRIBED
NOTES			TREATMENT
			FOLLOW UP

DATE	TIME	DOCTOR		CONTACT
REASON FOR VISIT		QUESTIONS		OUTCOME
				MEDICATION PERSCRIBED
NOTES				TREATMENT
				FOLLOW UP

DATE	TIME	DOCTOR		CONTACT
REASON FOR VISIT		QUESTIONS		OUTCOME
				MEDICATION PERSCRIBED
NOTES				TREATMENT
				FOLLOW UP

DATE	TIME	DOCTOR		CONTACT
REASON FOR VISIT		QUESTIONS		OUTCOME
				MEDICATION PERSCRIBED
NOTES				TREATMENT
				FOLLOW UP

DATE	TIME	DOCTOR		CONTACT
REASON FOR VISIT		QUESTIONS		OUTCOME
				MEDICATION PERSCRIBED
NOTES				TREATMENT
				FOLLOW UP

DATE	TIME	DOCTOR		CONTACT
REASON FOR VISIT		QUESTIONS		OUTCOME
				MEDICATION PERSCRIBED
NOTES				TREATMENT
				FOLLOW UP

DATE	TIME	DOCTOR		CONTACT
REASON FOR VISIT		QUESTIONS		OUTCOME
				MEDICATION PERSCRIBED
NOTES				TREATMENT
				FOLLOW UP

DATE	TIME	DOCTOR		CONTACT
REASON FOR VISIT		QUESTIONS		OUTCOME
				MEDICATION PERSCRIBED
NOTES				TREATMENT
				FOLLOW UP

DATE	TIME	DOCTOR		CONTACT
REASON FOR VISIT		QUESTIONS		OUTCOME
				MEDICATION PERSCRIBED
NOTES				TREATMENT
				FOLLOW UP

DATE	TIME	DOCTOR		CONTACT
REASON FOR VISIT		QUESTIONS		OUTCOME
				MEDICATION PERSCRIBED
NOTES				TREATMENT
				FOLLOW UP

DATE	TIME	DOCTOR		CONTACT
REASON FOR VISIT		QUESTIONS		OUTCOME
				MEDICATION PERSCRIBED
NOTES				TREATMENT
				FOLLOW UP

DATE	TIME	DOCTOR		CONTACT
REASON FOR VISIT		QUESTIONS		OUTCOME
				MEDICATION PERSCRIBED
NOTES				TREATMENT
				FOLLOW UP

DATE	TIME	DOCTOR		CONTACT
REASON FOR VISIT		QUESTIONS		OUTCOME
				MEDICATION PERSCRIBED
NOTES				TREATMENT
				FOLLOW UP

DATE	TIME	DOCTOR		CONTACT
REASON FOR VISIT		QUESTIONS		OUTCOME
				MEDICATION PERSCRIBED
NOTES				TREATMENT
				FOLLOW UP

DATE	TIME	DOCTOR		CONTACT
REASON FOR VISIT		QUESTIONS		OUTCOME
				MEDICATION PERSCRIBED
NOTES				TREATMENT
				FOLLOW UP

DATE	TIME	DOCTOR		CONTACT
REASON FOR VISIT		QUESTIONS		OUTCOME
				MEDICATION PERSCRIBED
NOTES				TREATMENT
				FOLLOW UP

DATE	TIME	DOCTOR		CONTACT
REASON FOR VISIT		QUESTIONS		OUTCOME
				MEDICATION PERSCRIBED
NOTES				TREATMENT
				FOLLOW UP

DATE	TIME	DOCTOR		CONTACT
REASON FOR VISIT		QUESTIONS		OUTCOME
				MEDICATION PERSCRIBED
NOTES				TREATMENT
				FOLLOW UP

DATE	TIME	DOCTOR		CONTACT
REASON FOR VISIT		QUESTIONS		OUTCOME
				MEDICATION PERSCRIBED
NOTES				TREATMENT
				FOLLOW UP

DATE	TIME	DOCTOR		CONTACT
REASON FOR VISIT		QUESTIONS		OUTCOME
				MEDICATION PERSCRIBED
NOTES				TREATMENT
				FOLLOW UP

DATE	TIME	DOCTOR		CONTACT
REASON FOR VISIT		QUESTIONS		OUTCOME
				MEDICATION PERSCRIBED
NOTES				TREATMENT
				FOLLOW UP

DATE	TIME	DOCTOR		CONTACT
REASON FOR VISIT		QUESTIONS		OUTCOME
				MEDICATION PERSCRIBED
NOTES				TREATMENT
				FOLLOW UP

DATE	TIME	DOCTOR		CONTACT
REASON FOR VISIT		QUESTIONS		OUTCOME
				MEDICATION PERSCRIBED
NOTES				TREATMENT
				FOLLOW UP

DATE	TIME	DOCTOR		CONTACT
REASON FOR VISIT		QUESTIONS		OUTCOME
				MEDICATION PERSCRIBED
NOTES				TREATMENT
				FOLLOW UP

DATE	TIME	DOCTOR		CONTACT
REASON FOR VISIT		QUESTIONS		OUTCOME
				MEDICATION PERSCRIBED
NOTES				TREATMENT
				FOLLOW UP

DATE	TIME	DOCTOR		CONTACT
REASON FOR VISIT		QUESTIONS		OUTCOME
				MEDICATION PERSCRIBED
NOTES				TREATMENT
				FOLLOW UP

DATE	TIME	DOCTOR		CONTACT
REASON FOR VISIT		QUESTIONS		OUTCOME
				MEDICATION PERSCRIBED
NOTES				TREATMENT
				FOLLOW UP

DATE	TIME	DOCTOR		CONTACT
REASON FOR VISIT		QUESTIONS		OUTCOME
				MEDICATION PERSCRIBED
NOTES				TREATMENT
				FOLLOW UP

DATE	TIME	DOCTOR	CONTACT

REASON FOR VISIT	QUESTIONS	OUTCOME
		MEDICATION PERSCRIBED

NOTES		TREATMENT
		FOLLOW UP

DATE	TIME	DOCTOR	CONTACT

REASON FOR VISIT	QUESTIONS	OUTCOME
		MEDICATION PERSCRIBED

NOTES		TREATMENT
		FOLLOW UP

DATE	TIME	DOCTOR	CONTACT

REASON FOR VISIT	QUESTIONS	OUTCOME
		MEDICATION PERSCRIBED

NOTES		TREATMENT
		FOLLOW UP

DATE	TIME	DOCTOR	CONTACT
REASON FOR VISIT		QUESTIONS	OUTCOME
			MEDICATION PERSCRIBED
NOTES			TREATMENT
			FOLLOW UP

DATE	TIME	DOCTOR	CONTACT
REASON FOR VISIT		QUESTIONS	OUTCOME
			MEDICATION PERSCRIBED
NOTES			TREATMENT
			FOLLOW UP

DATE	TIME	DOCTOR	CONTACT
REASON FOR VISIT		QUESTIONS	OUTCOME
			MEDICATION PERSCRIBED
NOTES			TREATMENT
			FOLLOW UP

DATE	TIME	DOCTOR	CONTACT
REASON FOR VISIT		QUESTIONS	OUTCOME
			MEDICATION PERSCRIBED
NOTES			TREATMENT
			FOLLOW UP

DATE	TIME	DOCTOR	CONTACT
REASON FOR VISIT		QUESTIONS	OUTCOME
			MEDICATION PERSCRIBED
NOTES			TREATMENT
			FOLLOW UP

DATE	TIME	DOCTOR	CONTACT
REASON FOR VISIT		QUESTIONS	OUTCOME
			MEDICATION PERSCRIBED
NOTES			TREATMENT
			FOLLOW UP

DATE	TIME	DOCTOR		CONTACT
REASON FOR VISIT		QUESTIONS		OUTCOME
				MEDICATION PERSCRIBED
NOTES				TREATMENT
				FOLLOW UP

DATE	TIME	DOCTOR		CONTACT
REASON FOR VISIT		QUESTIONS		OUTCOME
				MEDICATION PERSCRIBED
NOTES				TREATMENT
				FOLLOW UP

DATE	TIME	DOCTOR		CONTACT
REASON FOR VISIT		QUESTIONS		OUTCOME
				MEDICATION PERSCRIBED
NOTES				TREATMENT
				FOLLOW UP

DATE	TIME	DOCTOR		CONTACT
REASON FOR VISIT		QUESTIONS		OUTCOME
				MEDICATION PERSCRIBED
NOTES				TREATMENT
				FOLLOW UP

DATE	TIME	DOCTOR		CONTACT
REASON FOR VISIT		QUESTIONS		OUTCOME
				MEDICATION PERSCRIBED
NOTES				TREATMENT
				FOLLOW UP

DATE	TIME	DOCTOR		CONTACT
REASON FOR VISIT		QUESTIONS		OUTCOME
				MEDICATION PERSCRIBED
NOTES				TREATMENT
				FOLLOW UP

DATE	TIME	DOCTOR		CONTACT
REASON FOR VISIT		QUESTIONS		OUTCOME
				MEDICATION PERSCRIBED
NOTES				TREATMENT
				FOLLOW UP

DATE	TIME	DOCTOR		CONTACT
REASON FOR VISIT		QUESTIONS		OUTCOME
				MEDICATION PERSCRIBED
NOTES				TREATMENT
				FOLLOW UP

DATE	TIME	DOCTOR		CONTACT
REASON FOR VISIT		QUESTIONS		OUTCOME
				MEDICATION PERSCRIBED
NOTES				TREATMENT
				FOLLOW UP

DATE	TIME	DOCTOR		CONTACT
REASON FOR VISIT		QUESTIONS		OUTCOME
				MEDICATION PERSCRIBED
NOTES				TREATMENT
				FOLLOW UP

DATE	TIME	DOCTOR		CONTACT
REASON FOR VISIT		QUESTIONS		OUTCOME
				MEDICATION PERSCRIBED
NOTES				TREATMENT
				FOLLOW UP

DATE	TIME	DOCTOR		CONTACT
REASON FOR VISIT		QUESTIONS		OUTCOME
				MEDICATION PERSCRIBED
NOTES				TREATMENT
				FOLLOW UP

DATE	TIME	DOCTOR	CONTACT
REASON FOR VISIT		QUESTIONS	OUTCOME
			MEDICATION PERSCRIBED
NOTES			TREATMENT
			FOLLOW UP

DATE	TIME	DOCTOR	CONTACT
REASON FOR VISIT		QUESTIONS	OUTCOME
			MEDICATION PERSCRIBED
NOTES			TREATMENT
			FOLLOW UP

DATE	TIME	DOCTOR	CONTACT
REASON FOR VISIT		QUESTIONS	OUTCOME
			MEDICATION PERSCRIBED
NOTES			TREATMENT
			FOLLOW UP

DATE	TIME	DOCTOR	CONTACT
REASON FOR VISIT		QUESTIONS	OUTCOME
			MEDICATION PERSCRIBED
NOTES			TREATMENT
			FOLLOW UP

DATE	TIME	DOCTOR	CONTACT
REASON FOR VISIT		QUESTIONS	OUTCOME
			MEDICATION PERSCRIBED
NOTES			TREATMENT
			FOLLOW UP

DATE	TIME	DOCTOR	CONTACT
REASON FOR VISIT		QUESTIONS	OUTCOME
			MEDICATION PERSCRIBED
NOTES			TREATMENT
			FOLLOW UP

DATE	TIME	DOCTOR		CONTACT
REASON FOR VISIT		QUESTIONS		OUTCOME
				MEDICATION PERSCRIBED
NOTES				TREATMENT
				FOLLOW UP

DATE	TIME	DOCTOR		CONTACT
REASON FOR VISIT		QUESTIONS		OUTCOME
				MEDICATION PERSCRIBED
NOTES				TREATMENT
				FOLLOW UP

DATE	TIME	DOCTOR		CONTACT
REASON FOR VISIT		QUESTIONS		OUTCOME
				MEDICATION PERSCRIBED
NOTES				TREATMENT
				FOLLOW UP

DATE	TIME	DOCTOR		CONTACT
REASON FOR VISIT		QUESTIONS		OUTCOME
				MEDICATION PERSCRIBED
NOTES				TREATMENT
				FOLLOW UP

DATE	TIME	DOCTOR		CONTACT
REASON FOR VISIT		QUESTIONS		OUTCOME
				MEDICATION PERSCRIBED
NOTES				TREATMENT
				FOLLOW UP

DATE	TIME	DOCTOR		CONTACT
REASON FOR VISIT		QUESTIONS		OUTCOME
				MEDICATION PERSCRIBED
NOTES				TREATMENT
				FOLLOW UP

DATE	TIME	DOCTOR	CONTACT
REASON FOR VISIT		QUESTIONS	OUTCOME
			MEDICATION PERSCRIBED
NOTES			TREATMENT
			FOLLOW UP

DATE	TIME	DOCTOR	CONTACT
REASON FOR VISIT		QUESTIONS	OUTCOME
			MEDICATION PERSCRIBED
NOTES			TREATMENT
			FOLLOW UP

DATE	TIME	DOCTOR	CONTACT
REASON FOR VISIT		QUESTIONS	OUTCOME
			MEDICATION PERSCRIBED
NOTES			TREATMENT
			FOLLOW UP

DATE	TIME	DOCTOR		CONTACT
REASON FOR VISIT		QUESTIONS		OUTCOME
				MEDICATION PERSCRIBED
NOTES				TREATMENT
				FOLLOW UP

DATE	TIME	DOCTOR		CONTACT
REASON FOR VISIT		QUESTIONS		OUTCOME
				MEDICATION PERSCRIBED
NOTES				TREATMENT
				FOLLOW UP

DATE	TIME	DOCTOR		CONTACT
REASON FOR VISIT		QUESTIONS		OUTCOME
				MEDICATION PERSCRIBED
NOTES				TREATMENT
				FOLLOW UP

DATE	TIME	DOCTOR		CONTACT
REASON FOR VISIT		**QUESTIONS**		**OUTCOME**
				MEDICATION PERSCRIBED
NOTES				**TREATMENT**
				FOLLOW UP

DATE	TIME	DOCTOR		CONTACT
REASON FOR VISIT		**QUESTIONS**		**OUTCOME**
				MEDICATION PERSCRIBED
NOTES				**TREATMENT**
				FOLLOW UP

DATE	TIME	DOCTOR		CONTACT
REASON FOR VISIT		**QUESTIONS**		**OUTCOME**
				MEDICATION PERSCRIBED
NOTES				**TREATMENT**
				FOLLOW UP

DATE	TIME	DOCTOR		CONTACT
REASON FOR VISIT		QUESTIONS		OUTCOME
				MEDICATION PERSCRIBED
NOTES				TREATMENT
				FOLLOW UP

DATE	TIME	DOCTOR		CONTACT
REASON FOR VISIT		QUESTIONS		OUTCOME
				MEDICATION PERSCRIBED
NOTES				TREATMENT
				FOLLOW UP

DATE	TIME	DOCTOR		CONTACT
REASON FOR VISIT		QUESTIONS		OUTCOME
				MEDICATION PERSCRIBED
NOTES				TREATMENT
				FOLLOW UP

DATE	TIME	DOCTOR		CONTACT
REASON FOR VISIT		QUESTIONS		OUTCOME
				MEDICATION PERSCRIBED
NOTES				TREATMENT
				FOLLOW UP

DATE	TIME	DOCTOR		CONTACT
REASON FOR VISIT		QUESTIONS		OUTCOME
				MEDICATION PERSCRIBED
NOTES				TREATMENT
				FOLLOW UP

DATE	TIME	DOCTOR		CONTACT
REASON FOR VISIT		QUESTIONS		OUTCOME
				MEDICATION PERSCRIBED
NOTES				TREATMENT
				FOLLOW UP

DATE	TIME	DOCTOR		CONTACT
REASON FOR VISIT		QUESTIONS		OUTCOME
				MEDICATION PERSCRIBED
NOTES				TREATMENT
				FOLLOW UP

DATE	TIME	DOCTOR		CONTACT
REASON FOR VISIT		QUESTIONS		OUTCOME
				MEDICATION PERSCRIBED
NOTES				TREATMENT
				FOLLOW UP

DATE	TIME	DOCTOR		CONTACT
REASON FOR VISIT		QUESTIONS		OUTCOME
				MEDICATION PERSCRIBED
NOTES				TREATMENT
				FOLLOW UP

DATE	TIME	DOCTOR		CONTACT
REASON FOR VISIT		QUESTIONS		OUTCOME
				MEDICATION PERSCRIBED
NOTES				TREATMENT
				FOLLOW UP

DATE	TIME	DOCTOR		CONTACT
REASON FOR VISIT		QUESTIONS		OUTCOME
				MEDICATION PERSCRIBED
NOTES				TREATMENT
				FOLLOW UP

DATE	TIME	DOCTOR		CONTACT
REASON FOR VISIT		QUESTIONS		OUTCOME
				MEDICATION PERSCRIBED
NOTES				TREATMENT
				FOLLOW UP

DATE	TIME	DOCTOR		CONTACT
REASON FOR VISIT		QUESTIONS		OUTCOME
				MEDICATION PERSCRIBED
NOTES				TREATMENT
				FOLLOW UP

DATE	TIME	DOCTOR		CONTACT
REASON FOR VISIT		QUESTIONS		OUTCOME
				MEDICATION PERSCRIBED
NOTES				TREATMENT
				FOLLOW UP

DATE	TIME	DOCTOR		CONTACT
REASON FOR VISIT		QUESTIONS		OUTCOME
				MEDICATION PERSCRIBED
NOTES				TREATMENT
				FOLLOW UP

DATE	TIME	DOCTOR		CONTACT
REASON FOR VISIT		QUESTIONS		OUTCOME
				MEDICATION PERSCRIBED
NOTES				TREATMENT
				FOLLOW UP

DATE	TIME	DOCTOR		CONTACT
REASON FOR VISIT		QUESTIONS		OUTCOME
				MEDICATION PERSCRIBED
NOTES				TREATMENT
				FOLLOW UP

DATE	TIME	DOCTOR		CONTACT
REASON FOR VISIT		QUESTIONS		OUTCOME
				MEDICATION PERSCRIBED
NOTES				TREATMENT
				FOLLOW UP

DATE	TIME	DOCTOR		CONTACT
REASON FOR VISIT		QUESTIONS		OUTCOME
				MEDICATION PERSCRIBED
NOTES				TREATMENT
				FOLLOW UP

DATE	TIME	DOCTOR		CONTACT
REASON FOR VISIT		QUESTIONS		OUTCOME
				MEDICATION PERSCRIBED
NOTES				TREATMENT
				FOLLOW UP

DATE	TIME	DOCTOR		CONTACT
REASON FOR VISIT		QUESTIONS		OUTCOME
				MEDICATION PERSCRIBED
NOTES				TREATMENT
				FOLLOW UP

DATE	TIME	DOCTOR	CONTACT
REASON FOR VISIT		QUESTIONS	OUTCOME
			MEDICATION PERSCRIBED
NOTES			TREATMENT
			FOLLOW UP

DATE	TIME	DOCTOR	CONTACT
REASON FOR VISIT		QUESTIONS	OUTCOME
			MEDICATION PERSCRIBED
NOTES			TREATMENT
			FOLLOW UP

DATE	TIME	DOCTOR	CONTACT
REASON FOR VISIT		QUESTIONS	OUTCOME
			MEDICATION PERSCRIBED
NOTES			TREATMENT
			FOLLOW UP

DATE	TIME	DOCTOR	CONTACT

REASON FOR VISIT	QUESTIONS	OUTCOME
		MEDICATION PERSCRIBED

NOTES	TREATMENT
	FOLLOW UP

DATE	TIME	DOCTOR	CONTACT

REASON FOR VISIT	QUESTIONS	OUTCOME
		MEDICATION PERSCRIBED

NOTES	TREATMENT
	FOLLOW UP

DATE	TIME	DOCTOR	CONTACT

REASON FOR VISIT	QUESTIONS	OUTCOME
		MEDICATION PERSCRIBED

NOTES	TREATMENT
	FOLLOW UP

DATE	TIME	DOCTOR	CONTACT
REASON FOR VISIT		**QUESTIONS**	**OUTCOME**
			MEDICATION PERSCRIBED
NOTES			**TREATMENT**
			FOLLOW UP

DATE	TIME	DOCTOR	CONTACT
REASON FOR VISIT		**QUESTIONS**	**OUTCOME**
			MEDICATION PERSCRIBED
NOTES			**TREATMENT**
			FOLLOW UP

DATE	TIME	DOCTOR	CONTACT
REASON FOR VISIT		**QUESTIONS**	**OUTCOME**
			MEDICATION PERSCRIBED
NOTES			**TREATMENT**
			FOLLOW UP

DATE	TIME	DOCTOR	CONTACT
REASON FOR VISIT		QUESTIONS	OUTCOME
			MEDICATION PERSCRIBED
NOTES			TREATMENT
			FOLLOW UP

DATE	TIME	DOCTOR	CONTACT
REASON FOR VISIT		QUESTIONS	OUTCOME
			MEDICATION PERSCRIBED
NOTES			TREATMENT
			FOLLOW UP

DATE	TIME	DOCTOR	CONTACT
REASON FOR VISIT		QUESTIONS	OUTCOME
			MEDICATION PERSCRIBED
NOTES			TREATMENT
			FOLLOW UP

DATE	TIME	DOCTOR		CONTACT
REASON FOR VISIT		QUESTIONS		OUTCOME
				MEDICATION PERSCRIBED
NOTES				TREATMENT
				FOLLOW UP

DATE	TIME	DOCTOR		CONTACT
REASON FOR VISIT		QUESTIONS		OUTCOME
				MEDICATION PERSCRIBED
NOTES				TREATMENT
				FOLLOW UP

DATE	TIME	DOCTOR		CONTACT
REASON FOR VISIT		QUESTIONS		OUTCOME
				MEDICATION PERSCRIBED
NOTES				TREATMENT
				FOLLOW UP

DATE	TIME	DOCTOR		CONTACT
REASON FOR VISIT		QUESTIONS		OUTCOME
				MEDICATION PERSCRIBED
NOTES				TREATMENT
				FOLLOW UP

DATE	TIME	DOCTOR		CONTACT
REASON FOR VISIT		QUESTIONS		OUTCOME
				MEDICATION PERSCRIBED
NOTES				TREATMENT
				FOLLOW UP

DATE	TIME	DOCTOR		CONTACT
REASON FOR VISIT		QUESTIONS		OUTCOME
				MEDICATION PERSCRIBED
NOTES				TREATMENT
				FOLLOW UP

DATE	TIME	DOCTOR		CONTACT
REASON FOR VISIT		QUESTIONS		OUTCOME
				MEDICATION PERSCRIBED
NOTES				TREATMENT
				FOLLOW UP

DATE	TIME	DOCTOR		CONTACT
REASON FOR VISIT		QUESTIONS		OUTCOME
				MEDICATION PERSCRIBED
NOTES				TREATMENT
				FOLLOW UP

DATE	TIME	DOCTOR		CONTACT
REASON FOR VISIT		QUESTIONS		OUTCOME
				MEDICATION PERSCRIBED
NOTES				TREATMENT
				FOLLOW UP

DATE	TIME	DOCTOR		CONTACT
REASON FOR VISIT		QUESTIONS		OUTCOME
				MEDICATION PERSCRIBED
NOTES				TREATMENT
				FOLLOW UP

DATE	TIME	DOCTOR		CONTACT
REASON FOR VISIT		QUESTIONS		OUTCOME
				MEDICATION PERSCRIBED
NOTES				TREATMENT
				FOLLOW UP

DATE	TIME	DOCTOR		CONTACT
REASON FOR VISIT		QUESTIONS		OUTCOME
				MEDICATION PERSCRIBED
NOTES				TREATMENT
				FOLLOW UP

DATE	TIME	DOCTOR	CONTACT
REASON FOR VISIT		QUESTIONS	OUTCOME
			MEDICATION PERSCRIBED
NOTES			TREATMENT
			FOLLOW UP

DATE	TIME	DOCTOR	CONTACT
REASON FOR VISIT		QUESTIONS	OUTCOME
			MEDICATION PERSCRIBED
NOTES			TREATMENT
			FOLLOW UP

DATE	TIME	DOCTOR	CONTACT
REASON FOR VISIT		QUESTIONS	OUTCOME
			MEDICATION PERSCRIBED
NOTES			TREATMENT
			FOLLOW UP

Copyright © 2020 MPX2 Publishing Company
All Rights Reserved

Printed in Great Britain
by Amazon

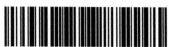
34954248R00070